A Practical Treatise on Smallpox
By George Henry Fox

PREFACE.

Whenever a physician is called to a case of suspected smallpox, he confronts a grave responsibility. If young or without special experience, he is apt to feel a sore need of assistance, and, although a book can never take the place of an experienced consultant, it is the object of the present work to render him as much aid as possible. The text aims to be practical rather than elaborate. The plates are reproductions of photographs from life, some of which have been obtained under great difficulty.

While many articles on variola have been illustrated by a few photographs of cases, mostly of the pustular type, this work is believed to be the first which has presented illustrations of the smallpox eruption in each of its successive stages. It is sincerely hoped that the reader will find it of service in familiarizing him with the peculiar features of the disease.

GEORGE HENRY FOX.

SMALLPOX.

CHAPTER I.

VARIOLA, or smallpox, is an acute, contagious disease, characterized by an eruption upon both the skin and mucous membrane, with constitutional symptoms of greater or less severity. The eruption presents successively a macular, papular, vesicular, and pustular stage, the pustules finally drying into crusts, which fall and leave the skin temporarily discolored. Where ulceration has occurred it is permanently scarred or pitted. The lesions of the mucous membrane appear upon those parts more or less exposed to the air,—the mouth and eyes, for example,—but in exceptional cases they may be found throughout the entire intestinal tract, and in the uterus and bladder. These lesions do not run a course similar to those observed upon the skin, but appear as red macules, which rapidly change into ulcerations, covered with a whitish pellicle. The ulcers are imbedded in the substance of the mucous membrane and are not as superficial as in cancrum oris. The constitutional symptoms are most prominent during the periods of invasion and pustulation.

There are various clinical forms of smallpox, which may be conveniently described as (1) discrete, (2) confluent, and (3) hemorrhagic, or malignant; and then, according to intensity, as (a) very mild, (b) mild, and (c) severe. The few purpuric spots seen in the severe discrete and the confluent forms are not of great significance, as they are generally due to a peculiar diathesis, and as a rule the patient recovers. The malignant form is almost invariably fatal.

The term discrete implies that the lesions are separate and distinct, not coalescent. If the lesions coalesce and form patches of various shapes and sizes, the eruption is called confluent. For the purpose of differentiating the various forms above mentioned, it is convenient to first trace a normal, unmodified case of smallpox from the initial symptoms to recovery, and then to consider the severe forms, and finally the rare and obscure forms of the disease.

Period of Incubation.—This extends from the date of exposure to the occurrence of clinical symptoms, a period usually lasting from twelve to fourteen days.

Period of Invasion.—The disease is usually ushered in by fever, with a distinct chill or chilly sensations, headache, neuralgia, and a general malaise. Frequently the first symptom is a distressing backache. This is located in the lumbar region, but it may be as high up as the lower angle of the scapula, or it may be sacral and extend down into the thighs. The backache is an important symptom when present, but it is not always on hand to help one out in the diagnosis. The backache of smallpox is not peculiar or distinctive, but it is its severity which attracts attention.

The headache is usually frontal and is an ache that is constant in character. The neuralgia is about the orbits, but may be facial, and is of a lancinating character.

The fever may precede the backache or it may follow. It may be at first a rise of only a

4

degree or two, or it may jump to 104° F., or as high as 106° F. The latter is most frequently seen in neurasthenic subjects and in children. The pulse rises in frequency and in tension.

In children a convulsion not infrequently ushers in the disease. At this time convulsions are of little significance, but late in the disease they are of serious import. There are other constitutional symptoms, such as loss of appetite, vomiting, muscular pains, a dry, coated tongue, and at times an active delirium.

The face is congested and swollen. The eyes are injected and present a bleared appearance, but the watery or weeping condition seen in measles is usually absent. The nose is dry, and a sore throat is not uncommon. Epistaxis is frequent.

A very important symptom which sometimes occurs in this stage is a cutaneous efflorescence, which may resemble urticaria, scarlet fever, or measles. This latter resemblance is very close and often leads to diagnostic error. The efflorescence occurs most frequently in the young, and also in vaccinated adults. In some epidemics it is not at all uncommon, but as a rule it is rare.

The duration of the stage of invasion varies from two to four days. Usually it is about three days.

Period of Eruption.—Late on the third day or early on the fourth the eruption makes its appearance, and the constitutional symptoms subside to a certain extent.

The rash appears first on the confined and moist portions of the skin or in irritated parts,—under a blister, for instance, which may have been applied for the backache. Normally, it is first seen upon the forehead at the hair-line, then behind the ears and down the tender part of the neck. It gradually extends down the trunk and arms, the hands and lower extremities being affected last. The eruption generally takes from twenty-four to thirty-six hours to cover the entire body. The best location to observe the rash for diagnostic purposes is on the back, where it cannot be obscured by scratching and where the warmth of the body causes the mildest congestion to appear at its best. The exposed parts are usually ill adapted for study of the rash, being obscured by the swelling and congestion of the face and by more or less dirt or staining of the hands.

The rash consists first of small round or oval, rose-colored macules, which seem to be in the skin, coming up from beneath it, as it were. They disappear readily on pressure or on tension of the skin. When coalescence occurs, the lesions may resemble the blotches of measles. The macule at this stage is about from one-eighth to one-fourth of an inch in diameter, and its color is of an intense red which shows well at night, even by the light of a match. In less than twenty-four hours the centre of the macule becomes hard; and as this hardness increases, the lesion gradually rises above the skin. It is now changing into the papular stage. The macular stage lasts usually from eight to twenty-four hours.

The papules continue to increase slowly in size, the apex becoming flattened or indented in some lesions. While this change is going on the redness of the macule forms an areola about the hard portion or central papule. This areola tends to get smaller as the papule gets larger, and at last is completely lost.

If the pulp of the finger is passed over the papule, especially in its early stage, the latter seems to roll beneath it, giving the sensation of a small shot buried in the skin. When the papule is fully developed, the surrounding skin is put on the stretch, and the rolling sensation is lost, but the papule is so dense and hard that it is frequently described as "shotty." The papule of varicella and of acne is not so dense and resisting as the papule of variola. The fully-developed papule in smallpox is rarely surrounded by a halo of congestion as it is in varicella, but in the modified form of smallpox this is not infrequently the case. The papule always arises from the centre of its halo like a bull's eye, whereas in chicken-pox it arises from within the circumference, but not always in the centre. The halo of congestion in chicken-pox is always very broad and extensive, and is best seen upon the back. When a halo is present in smallpox it is very narrow and insignificant. The papule is usually fully developed in twenty-four hours.

At the end of another twenty-four or thirty-six hours the apex of the papule shows a further change. It appears to be transformed from a solid to a fluid. The color also changes as the fluid increases, and the lesion appears bluish or purplish. The fluid continues to increase in amount until the papule is converted into a little blister or vesicle. As the change is going on, the height of the papule grows less and less, and when vesiculation is complete we have a broad, flat, umbilicated vesicle with a firm, dense base. To the touch these vesicles are firm and resisting, and the membranous covering is not easily broken, unless macerated by the perspiration due to heavy flannels.

The vesicle is divided irregularly by little bands, or septa, which permit only a portion of the fluid to escape when one is punctured. Vesiculation is usually complete about the third day, and the stage generally lasts three days. It may be stated here that the reckoning in smallpox is usually from the appearance of the rash. The period of incubation and invasion are considered in reckoning the length of illness, but in descriptions of smallpox it is considered best to state the day of the eruption, and not of the disease.

There is an old and oft-repeated statement that a uniform rash is a characteristic of smallpox and that a mixed rash indicates chicken-pox. This deserves to be promptly refuted. It is most unusual to find a case of smallpox with its eruption all in one stage. While it is a well known fact that chicken-pox runs a hasty course,—so that in from one to two days we may have macules, papules, vesicles, and even crusts,—in smallpox this is not likely to occur, as the disease never runs such a rapid course. In the early stage we may see macules changing into papules on the head and the neck, while there are simply macules on the trunk. Later in the disease the eruption may be vesicular on the head while still papular on the body. When vesiculation is complete, we have the distinct umbilicated appearance that has long been recognized as a characteristic of smallpox. The vesicles are broad, firm, flat, and hard, and are invariably indented or umbilicated.

It is not until the stage of vesiculation that the constitutional symptoms diminish to a marked degree. In fact it is considered one of the landmarks of the disease for the fever curve to show a decline at this time.

Late in the fifth or early in the sixth day the vesicle begins to assume a cloudy or yellowish hue, which denotes the commencement of pustulation. The fluid continues to grow more yellow, and about the time that it has assumed a dense straw color the umbilication begins to disappear, so that in from one to three days the pustule loses its indented appearance and becomes globular in form. To the touch it appears to involve as much of the skin below the surface as it is high above it. It is during the stage of pustulation that the surrounding skin becomes swollen and œdematous, with an area of redness about the pustules giving the appearance of a bull's eye. It is also during the pustular stage that the constitutional symptoms become more intense and the fever rises in proportion to the severity of the attack. The pustules are fully matured about the eighth day of the eruption.

During the pustular stage the affection of the mucous membranes reaches its height. The eyelids, lips, and nose are often tremendously swollen. The tongue swells and deglutition becomes impossible. The voice is husky, and is sometimes lost, owing to the swelling of the glottis.

About the ninth or tenth day of the rash another change appears in the pustule. In mild cases this change sometimes takes place several days earlier. In the centre of the pustule is observed a small, darker spot, which gradually grows larger. The membrane of the pustule becomes shriveled, and the little, dark spot continues to get larger and darker until it involves the entire area of the pustule. This is the drying stage, during which the fluid part of the pustule is absorbed, leaving the solid part behind to be exfoliated in the form of a crust. It is during this stage that, owing to the softening of its membranous covering, the pustule is broken by the movements of the patient or the contact of rough bed-linen. The pustules of the face are usually the first ones broken, and an ulceration frequently occurs which destroys the true skin and results in a pit or scar. Pustules do not rupture spontaneously and discharge their contents. Dessication lasts usually from five to twenty days, the exposed parts being the first to dry and shed their crusts. On the palms and soles the dessicated débris is left deeply buried in the skin, and often has to be removed by the aid of a lancet or other instrument. Sometimes there is a pustule under the nail, and the removal of the kernel or seed is quite painful, though necessary.

The crust is usually thin, of a light yellowish-brown tint, but slightly adherent, and is shed or picked off without discomfort. The spot where the crust has been is of a deep purplish hue, and the many little stains here and there give the patient a peculiar spotted appearance, which in time disappears, except where the ulceration has left a pit or cicatrix. The pit soon loses its color and becomes of a whitish hue.

As dessication proceeds the constitutional symptoms decline, the appetite returns, and the patient gains strength.

Complications.—Sepsis is the one generally to be expected, and this may assume any form from a local affection, such as a furuncle, to a general septicæmia. Furunculosis is frequent and is often annoying, and no sooner is one boil healed than others follow. Bed-sores are also frequent if proper care is not used to prevent them. Bronchitis from the affection of the mucous membranes may occur. When simple, this can be handled easily; but when general pneumonia results, death is inevitable in the weakened condition of the patient. Ulcers and opacities of the cornea, laryngitis and croup (the latter generally fatal), zoster, sciatica, nephritis and gastritis, are all frequent complications, especially in severe cases.

Confluent Smallpox.—In this form the vesicles coalesce or run together, forming variously shaped and sized blisters, which as pustulation proceeds are usually ruptured in some manner and become infected, forming large, thick scabs with extensive ulceration underneath. The inability to properly cleanse such cases causes a very fetid odor to be given off and makes the patient an exceedingly difficult one to treat.

In the mild confluent form the disease is similar to the discrete form only that several lesions coalesce. In the severe confluent form the coalescence is extensive and large blisters are formed. The swelling about them is intense, and with the extensive sepsis the patient rarely survives. The swelling of the face and extremities is sometimes enormous, and the suffering is so severe as to make death a welcome visitor.

Confluent smallpox runs a course similar to that of the other forms, except that it is not as rapid as the third and is usually more severe than the first.

Hemorrhagic Smallpox.—This is recognized as the malignant form of variola, and is rapidly fatal in most cases. It runs its course precipitately, and at times most unexpectedly,—sometimes killing the patient in a few hours and in other cases not completing its career until the fourth or fifth day. Hemorrhages may come on suddenly and the patient expire before any rash appears. In one case an efflorescence appeared and so closely resembled scarlet fever that it was mistaken for it. Suddenly hemorrhages set in, and within six hours the patient was dead. There was a question at the time as to whether the case was malignant scarlet fever or malignant smallpox. Later a room-mate came down with a typical case of smallpox and helped to clear the doubt. The hemorrhage usually occurs as the disease changes from vesiculation into pustulation.

The severity of the hemorrhagic form of the disease is shown by the rapidity with which it passes through the various stages. Macules appear, and within a few hours rapidly change into papules, which almost as rapidly change into pustules; and before pustulation is complete hemorrhage occurs, and death quickly follows. It is not unusual in these cases for the disease to run its course in from twenty-four to thirty-six hours. In many, severe constitutional symptoms mark the onset, hemorrhages occur immediately, and death results before the rash appears. The hemorrhages are from the mucous membrane of the eyes, nose, and mouth, and from the anal, vaginal, and urethral orifices, the membrane swelling enormously. Hemorrhage occurring in the skin causes it to become raised and of a livid purple or bluish tint. The eyes seem to bulge as if about to drop from the orbital cavity. On the abdomen the hemorrhage is beneath the skin, causing raised lesions with a sharp border and a flattened top, feeling dense and firm to the touch. In the peritoneum the hemorrhages are extensive.

The constitutional symptoms in this severe form are typhoidal in character. The mind appears at ease, quietly passing into a comatose state. The countenance is pinched and sunken, and the skin is dusky and purplish. The eyes appear bloodshot and listless. The breathing is rapid and superficial. The delirium is of a quiet character, and death comes as a most welcome termination.

CASE I.—McD. Admitted to the hospital with a high fever (106.4° F.) and complaining of sore throat. One hour after admission there was noticed a very intense red rash, eyes bloodshot, and patient stupid. Patient isolated for scarlet fever. Hemorrhages came from eyes, nose, and mouth. Vomited blood in large quantities. Purplish spots appeared on the skin and spread rapidly over the whole cutaneous surface. Three hours after admission the patient died.

CASE II.—The patient, J. H., attended the funeral of a relative in New Jersey. Ten days afterwards he received a letter stating that the person had died of smallpox, but that they desired the matter to be kept secret. Feeling nervous, he got vaccinated. Three days from the receipt of the letter he did not return to work after his lunch, and complained of feeling weary. Went to bed, telling his wife to call him at four o'clock, as he had an important engagement. At half-past three his wife went to call him, and found him bleeding profusely. She called a neighboring doctor, who notified the Board of Health. The health inspector called at five P.M. Patient unconscious; face dark and dusky; eyeballs bulging and blood oozing from them. Hemorrhage from nose and mouth. Vomited a large quantity of dark, coagulated material. Pulseless at both wrists. Temperature 108° F., by rectum. Diagnosis, hemorrhagic variola. Ordered patient removed. Ambulance arrived at 7.15, just after the patient had died. No autopsy.

Through the courtesy of Dr. A. H. Doty, the following cases may be quoted. They were reported to the Health Department of New York City with a diagnosis of malignant hemorrhagic smallpox.

CASE I.—Mr. J. F., aged forty-four years. Removed to Reception Hospital on suspicion of typhus fever, December 8, 1893, when the following history was obtained: Patient was taken ill on December 3. On the following day, December 4, great weakness was experienced. Gradually became worse. Epistaxis, etc. On December 7 an eruption appeared. On December 8 the patient presented the following appearance: Face uniformly red, or of a dusky hue, and swollen; on close examination a faintly papular condition was apparent. Over chest, abdomen, and extremities was found a profuse papular eruption, of a very dusky or violet-colored hue. On the abdomen some of the papules had coalesced. Papules were noticeable on the hands and feet, particularly on the palms. On the inner surface of the thighs the entire skin presented the appearance of a scarlatinous eruption, although darker in color. Pressure on the surface did not leave a white streak or spot typical of scarlet fever. In some parts of the body papules were found which were almost black. At this time, December 8, there was no evidence of vesication. On December 9, the third day of the eruption, the latter presented no particular change in its appearance or progress. It still remained papular. Intense depression and delirium were present. At 3 P.M., December 9, the patient was removed to North Brothers Island. On December 10, the fourth day of the eruption, a few vesicles appeared for the first time. These formed slowly about the lower part of the abdomen and thighs. At these sites were four or five typical umbilications. On December 11, the fifth day of the eruption, many more umbilications were found. The patient became rapidly worse, and died on the following day, December 12.

CASE II.—Mr. F. S., aged twenty-four years. Removed to Reception Hospital on suspicion of typhus fever. On December 8 the appearance of this case was similar to Case I., inasmuch as the face was swollen and presented an erysipelatous appearance, although the color was more of a dusky hue. Large erythematous patches, suggestive of scarlet fever, were found covering different parts of the body. The same condition was present in this case as was noticed in Case I.,—i.e., the color of the patches was darker than in scarlet fever, and when the finger was drawn over the patch it did not leave a white line. No patches were found on the arms; but at these sites were dark, almost black, papules, which slowly became vesicular and umbilicated. The eruption was confluent on the upper part of the thighs and the face, and the patient died on December 8.

9

CASE III.—Mr. P. B., aged twenty-six years. Removed to Reception Hospital, December 16, 1893, on suspicion of typhus fever. On December 17 he presented the following appearance: The face and the entire trunk and upper portions of the thighs and shoulders presented an eruption which could easily have been mistaken for scarlet fever. The eruption was dotted with dark or black papules; some vesicles were noticed on the trunk. The eruption on the thighs was shotty and umbilicated and quite characteristic of variola. The face presented the same appearance as in Cases I. and II. On the legs and forearms, where the general redness was not present, the eruption had hardly gone beyond the macular stage, but was very dark,—almost black. As in the other cases, the finger drawn across left no white mark. It was stated that epistaxis had occurred. The patient became rapidly worse, without much change in the eruption, and died on December 17.

CASE IV.—Mr. L. R., lawyer, aged forty-three years. Removed from boarding-house, December 24, 1893, to Reception Hospital. Seen at home previous to removal, December 24. Patient felt badly on December 17. On December 20 was quite ill; pains in different parts of the body; nausea and vomiting. This condition continued until December 23, when an eruption appeared. Diagnosis, scarlet fever. On December 24, with the exception of the legs and forearms, the entire body and face was involved in a general eruption resembling scarlet fever. However, as in the preceding cases, it was of a darker hue than that found in scarlet fever, and pressure upon the skin made no impression so far as changing its color. Over the legs and forearm was distributed a profuse papular eruption, very dark in color. On other parts of the body were scattered some dark or almost black papules, with a few vesicles; typical umbilication was also present in some. A few small vesicles were noticed on the nose. These had the appearance of inflamed follicles, and were not as dark colored as the rest. The conjunctivæ were very much congested, and the membrane of the mouth was so much swollen that it was impossible to examine the throat. Hematemesis was present, also great prostration from the outset. The patient died on December 25.

CHAPTER II.

THERE are few diseases the prompt recognition of which is of greater importance to the physician than variola. On the one hand, failure to recognize the disease may subject the family of the patient and the community at large to the danger of contagion, and thus even be the starting-point of a widespread epidemic; on the other hand, to pronounce a case smallpox when it is not, entails so much needless pain and anxiety that the physician guilty of so grave an error merits the severe condemnation which will certainly be visited upon him.

The recognition of a case of smallpox may be simple, difficult, or even impossible, depending on the case and on the stage of the disease. In general the disease is readily recognized when the case is typical and the eruption has reached the vesicular or pustular stage. The diagnosis is difficult in atypical and complicated cases. It is impossible with any degree of positiveness in most cases in the pre-eruption period,—the stage of invasion.

The initial symptoms of smallpox resemble the first symptoms of so many infectious fevers that it is only through a consideration of the prevalence of an epidemic and the opportunities for infection in a given case that the physician may be put on his guard. It is important in this connection to notice whether the patient has been successfully vaccinated within a recent period. The physician who during the prevalence of an epidemic finds an unvaccinated subject suffering from a febrile disease of acute onset, with severe lumbar and dorsal pains, may, in the absence of definite symptoms pointing to some other disease, suspect smallpox; but a positive diagnosis at this stage is, of course, impossible.

Prodromal Rashes.—The occurrence of the prodromal rashes, the roseola variolosa,—a more or less diffuse scarlatiniform, morbillic, or urticarial rash which may appear on the second day of the fever,—has a certain diagnostic value; but this roseola occurs in only a small percentage of the cases, and, unfortunately, sometimes appears in other acute toxæmic conditions,—typhoid, for instance. The scarlatiniform rash may lead to a diagnosis of scarlet fever and the morbillic roseola be mistaken for measles; but these diseases would be excluded by the absence of the angina and the strawberry tongue of scarlatina in the one case and of the catarrhal symptoms of measles in the other, aside from other considerations. The appearance of the eruption on the second day of scarlatina is followed by a marked defervescence, while the scarlet rash of smallpox is not accompanied by any change in the temperature curve. The eruption in measles occurs on the fourth day of the illness, a circumstance which alone suffices to differentiate it from the morbilliform roseola of smallpox. The characteristic and pathognomonic "Koplik spots" on the buccal mucous membrane in measles are, of course, absent in smallpox. Furthermore, these prodromal eruptions of variola are of extremely evanescent character and usually disappear within eight or ten hours.

Of somewhat greater diagnostic value in this stage is the appearance of small hemorrhages, or petechiæ, varying in size from a pin's head to a pea, in the brachial and crural triangles of Simon. This form of prodromal eruption, however, is extremely rare, and, it may be added, is of grave prognostic significance, as it is usually the precursor of hemorrhagic smallpox.

Meningitis.—The intense headache, vertigo, delirium, and coma of meningitis, especially meningitis of the convexity without localizing symptoms, may be mistaken for severe prodromal symptoms of smallpox. As a rule, pulse and respiration are slow in meningitis, while in smallpox respiration and pulse are both markedly rapid.

Cerebro-spinal Meningitis.—In cerebro-spinal meningitis, in which an erythematous or purpuric rash appears, the difficulties of diagnosis are often such as tax the skill of the most expert clinician. It is important to remember that the rash of cerebro-spinal meningitis usually develops gradually or in successive crops, and that its distribution over the cutaneous surface is irregular, while the eruption of smallpox makes its complete appearance within the space of a few hours and is localized chiefly on the face and extremities. The stiffness at the back of the neck and the retraction of the head are symptoms that do not belong to smallpox.

Septicæmia and Pyæmia.—Acute septicæmic and pyæmic conditions in which there are hemorrhagic and bullous lesions in the skin sometimes present grave difficulties in making a differential diagnosis from smallpox. In general, however, a careful elucidation of the history of the case will bring out some points that serve for differentiation.

It must be admitted, however, that the diagnosis between cryptogenetic septicæmia and hemorrhagic smallpox is sometimes impossible *intra vitam*. A case of this kind may be cited which occurred in New York during the epidemic last year. A woman of thirty, not vaccinated since childhood, living in a house adjoining one from which a case of smallpox had been removed, was reported to the authorities as a possible case of smallpox. It was the sixth day of her illness, which had begun abruptly with headache, backache, vomiting, and fever. On the third day of the illness there was a profuse hemorrhage from the uterus, and thereafter metrorrhagia was almost constant. On the fourth day a scarlatiniform eruption was noticed on the legs and abdomen. The rash rapidly extended and was soon interspersed with hemorrhagic points. When seen on the evening of the sixth day the patient was semi-comatose. The skin was literally covered with a dusky scarlet rash in which were noted countless hemorrhagic macules, from a pin-point to a bean in size. The conjunctivæ bulbi were chemotic, the tongue was swollen, and the fauces were deeply congested. The post-mortem examination made the following morning, six hours after death, revealed a septic endometritis, and streptococci were cultivated from the blood and the peritoneal serum.

Grippe.—An attack of grippe may simulate the early symptoms of smallpox very closely. The onset may be sudden, the muscular pains severe, the pyrexia decided, the general prostration as marked as in smallpox. In grippe, however, the muscular pains are, as a rule, more general than in smallpox, there is rarely profuse sweating, and symptoms referable to the respiratory tract soon develop, if indeed they are not present from the beginning.

Rheumatism.—The severe lumbar and sacral pains of smallpox have been mistaken for rheumatism, but such an error can be made only where the use of the clinical thermometer is unknown. A febrile movement in lumbago is absent or but slight, while in smallpox the pyrexia is usually pronounced.

Typhoid and Typhus.—Typhoid and typhus fevers have at times been confounded with smallpox. But errors of this kind can be made only where the history of the case is completely ignored. In typhus, it is true, the eruption, petechial and almost papular in character, may suggest hemorrhagic smallpox; but the eruption of typhus rarely appears before the fourth or fifth day of the illness and is located chiefly on the trunk, sparing the face. The rash of malignant smallpox develops usually on the third or even the second day of the illness and is not limited to the trunk.

Upon the appearance of the rash in a typical case of smallpox the febrile diseases with which it is most frequently confounded are measles and varicella. It is interesting to note that until the time of Sydenham, in the latter part of the seventeenth century, measles and smallpox were regarded as manifestations of the same disease, and that the Vienna school of dermatologists, even to this day, insists on the etiological unity of variola and varicella.

Measles.—As a matter of fact the early papular eruption of measles bears a considerable resemblance to the first stage of the eruption of smallpox. In both the eruption is noted first in the face. In smallpox, however, the papules have a firm, "shotty" feeling on palpation, while in measles they are smooth and velvety to the touch. In measles the eruption, viewed at a little distance, seems to present a distinctly corymbose or crescentic grouping, an arrangement which is absent in smallpox. The eruption of smallpox appears at the end of the third day, that of measles on the fourth day. The temperature in smallpox undergoes a rapid defervescence upon the appearance of the rash, while in measles it continues to rise after the eruption appears. The pronounced pain in the back is absent in measles, while the very marked catarrhal symptoms, coryza, conjunctivitis, etc., are lacking in smallpox. The subsequent course of the eruption will leave no room for doubt, since within twenty-four hours the papules of smallpox will have developed into characteristic vesicles.

Varicella.—In varicella the stage of invasion is usually much shorter than in smallpox, the prostration less marked, and the lumbar pains of the latter disease are absent. The eruption in varicella comes out in successive crops and runs a shorter course, so that lesions in various stages of development may be seen side by side. The temperature does not necessarily fall on the appearance of the eruption, and there may be a more or less marked rise with each fresh crop of vesicles, the temperature curve presenting thus a remittent character. The eruption itself presents marked differences in the character and the course of the individual lesions, as well as in their distribution. The clear vesicles shoot up from the surface, as it were, without warning; or there may be for a brief period only a circumscribed erythema like that which usually precedes the appearance of an urticarial wheal. The vesicles of varicella have usually a somewhat obtusely conical shape, while those of smallpox are distinctly hemispherical. The characteristic umbilication of the smallpox vesicle is wanting in varicella. It is true the varicella vesicle often shows a depression at its apex; but this false umbilication, as it is called, is due to the rupture of the vesicle and the escape of some of its fluid or to a partial drying of its watery contents, and occurs only after the vesicle has existed for some time. The vesicle of varicella appears much more superficial in its seat, and its roof is much thinner, so that it ruptures readily. Very moderate pressure with the finger suffices to break it. When ruptured in this way the vesicle usually collapses completely, contrasting in this respect with the smallpox vesicle, from which, owing to the multilocular character of the lesion, all the fluid does not escape.

In varicella the distribution of the lesions over the surface is far more erratic than in smallpox. The very decided tendency to grouping of lesions upon the face and about the wrists so characteristic of smallpox does not occur in varicella, in which the vesicles may appear even more extensively on the trunk than upon the face. In varicella the palms and the soles, except in infants, are almost never affected; while in smallpox these regions are practically never exempt. It is true that in the extraordinarily mild cases of smallpox, such as have constituted the majority of cases during the past two years throughout the West, lesions may or may not be present on the palms and soles; but in the severe and moderately severe cases, such as have characterized the recent epidemic in New York, the soles and especially the palms have practically without exception shown the lesions. The localization of smallpox lesions on the palms and soles deserves far more emphasis than is generally accorded it in the textbooks, many of which even fail to mention it all. It may be put down as a safe rule that a case showing an extensive eruption of vesicles or pustules, however suspicious in other respects, is not smallpox if the palms and soles are free.

Acne.—Among the skin diseases proper there are a few whose appearance upon hasty examination may occasion some confusion with smallpox. Acne pustulosa presents only a superficial resemblance to variola, but in cases where it is accidentally associated with an acute febrile disease, like grippe, for instance, it may give rise to some diagnostic difficulty. In these cases, however, inquiry will develop the fact that the acne lesions have been present before the inception of the febrile disease; and the presence of comedos, the limitation of the lesions to the face, chest, and back, together with the absence of any lesions on the palms and soles, will serve to exclude smallpox.

Impetigo Contagiosa.—In impetigo contagiosa there might under similar circumstances be a momentary doubt as to the nature of the illness. Impetigo lesions have no typical distribution on the surface, the mucous membranes are always exempt; the vesicle itself is extremely superficial, ruptures very readily, and is at once replaced by a crust, so that lesions in various stages, vesicles, pustules, and crusts may always be seen at the same time.

Zoster.—Zoster is, as a rule, readily distinguished by the definite grouping of the lesions in the tract supplied by one or more nerves, its asymmetrical distribution, and the more or less severe neuralgic pain that precedes or accompanies the eruption. It must be remembered, however, that in zoster, in addition to the typical grouped lesions, there are occasionally seen a few isolated vesico-pustules scattered promiscuously over the entire surface; and the difficulty of diagnosis may be increased by the occurrence of a moderate temperature movement. In these cases, to which attention was first called by Teneson, the history of the case, the presence of characteristic herpetic groups, and the evolution and course of the individual lesions will suffice to clear the diagnosis.

Drug Eruptions.—The ingestion of bromides, iodides, and quinine is sometimes followed by an eruption which may create some confusion in diagnosis. In general the drug eruptions may be distinguished by the absence of fever and of the subjective symptoms of smallpox. The bromide and the iodide acne never occur on the palms and soles, where there are no sebaceous glands, and the lesions lack the evolution and course of the variolous eruption. The erythematous and purpuric eruption of quinine may be confused with the hemorrhagic form of smallpox; but here, too, the history of the course of the illness and the absence of fever will obviate the difficulty.

Syphilis.—Of all the diseases of the skin it is the pustular syphilide which most resembles the lesions of smallpox. Dermatologists and experts in variola are agreed that the pustular syphilide may be absolutely indistinguishable from smallpox so far as the appearance and distribution of the lesions is concerned. Furthermore, the pustular syphilide is frequently accompanied by a decided febrile movement. The differential diagnosis can be made in these cases only by the closest inquiry into the history of the case and by careful observation of the course of the disease. The characteristic history of an acute illness of short duration followed by a remission on the appearance of the eruption will of course be wanting in syphilis. The syphilitic eruption is more sluggish in its evolution as well as in the course of its subsequent changes; and though there may be lesions of syphilis on the mucous membrane of the mouth, they will lack the characteristic appearance of the vesicles and pustules of smallpox in this region. The palms and soles are not apt to show any lesions in this form of syphilis; and finally some other forms of syphilitic manifestation are very often present in this polymorphic disease to give the clue to the real nature of the eruption.

In conclusion, the fact should be emphasized that there are cases of smallpox of so mild a character, with general symptoms so slight and eruption so sparse and ill-defined, as to make a positive diagnosis extremely difficult. It is a good plan to employ vaccination in such cases as a test. Within three or four days the experienced observer will be able to determine whether the vaccination is successful or not; a negative result will of course have but a moderate value, but a positive result will serve to definitely exclude the diagnosis of smallpox. In all cases of doubt, whether before or after the eruption has appeared, the physician owes it to himself not less than to the patient and the community to frankly explain to the patient or his family the difficulty in arriving at a diagnosis, and to express his suspicions that the case may be one of smallpox. It need hardly be said that such a case should be as strictly isolated as if the diagnosis of smallpox were already established.

CHAPTER III.

IN the treatment of smallpox the therapeutic measures employed must necessarily vary with the severity of the disease and the condition of the patient in its successive stages. No remedy or plan of treatment will apply to all cases and at all times. As in the other exanthemata, there are cases of variola in which the disease runs so mild a course that a little nursing or simple attention to the personal comfort of the patient is all that is absolutely necessary. Such cases occur in those who have already had the disease,—for a second attack of smallpox must always be considered as a possibility, although it is a more rare occurrence than some writers would lead us to believe. Such cases also occur and with the greatest frequency in those who have been rendered more or less immune by a previous vaccination. But mild cases of smallpox may also occur among the unvaccinated; and in the present epidemic I have noted a few cases where, in spite of the lack of any protection from vaccination, the eruption and other symptoms of the disease were quite as mild as in some cases of so-called varioloid, or smallpox modified by previous vaccination.

In contrast with these cases which require no special medical treatment, there are others of marked severity with unexpected complications which tax the physician's skill to its utmost capacity. Still another class of cases, fortunately rare in most epidemics, are those to which the name of variola maligna has been given, and in which medical treatment seems to be almost as unnecessary as in the mild cases, since all attempts to avert a fatal termination have so far proved utterly futile.

In the successive stages of a typical case of variola a marked change in the character of the treatment is demanded both by the peculiarities of the eruption and the accompanying general symptoms. Instead of considering the various types of variola from a therapeutic stand-point, therefore, it would seem more practical to discuss in their natural order those measures which are adapted to the successive stages of the disease, beginning with the

Period of Incubation.—During this period, which extends from the date of infection to the appearance of the earliest symptoms of the disease, treatment is rarely demanded, since in the great majority of cases the outbreak of the disease is a surprise, and in no case can it be positively known that a patient has smallpox until the initial symptoms appear, and often not until the characteristic eruption has developed. In many instances, however, it is quite certain that an individual has been exposed to the contagion of variola; and when such a one happens to be unvaccinated, or has not been vaccinated in recent years, the assumption is strong that the disease may have been contracted and will manifest itself in due time.

The question as to whether vaccination can have any notable effect in modifying the course of variola when performed after a person has been exposed to and has

19

contracted the disease is one concerning which a considerable difference of opinion is expressed by modern writers. While some contend that even if vaccination fails to prevent the development of variola it is quite certain to modify its severity, others claim that it can be of no more advantage than locking the barn after a horse has been stolen.

The precise effect which vaccination during the stage of incubation may exert upon the subsequent course of the disease is very difficult to determine in one or even a small number of cases, since it is almost impossible to predict in any given case what the severity of the disease will be. In the opinion of Curschmann it is very doubtful whether vaccination can even render the course of smallpox milder. He states that in many instances where vaccination has been performed after exposure to smallpox infection the pustules of vaccinia and variola have been seen developing side by side, the former having apparently no effect upon the latter. In the opinion of Welsh, on the other hand, vaccination after infection often modifies the disease, and not infrequently prevents it altogether. He believes that when vaccinia has advanced to the stage of the formation of an areola around the vesicle, about the eighth day, it begins to exert its prophylactic power against smallpox; and as the period of incubation in variola is usually twelve days or more, an early vaccination may exert its protective influence in advance of the time when the variolous eruption should appear.

Welsh reports one hundred and ninety-four cases of vaccination performed during the stage of incubation, in which thirty-eight were perfectly protected against smallpox, sixteen almost perfectly protected, thirty-one protected to a well-marked degree, thirty partially protected, and seventy-nine were unprotected.

Of these one hundred and ninety-four cases the death-rate was 12.90 among those vaccinated early in the stage of incubation; it was 40.98 among those vaccinated from one to seven days before the eruption of smallpox appeared; while among the unvaccinated cases the death-rate amounted to fifty-eight per cent.

As it is well known that a secondary vaccination runs its course more rapidly than a primary one, it is evident that if an exposed patient has been already vaccinated a secondary vaccination is more apt to exert a protective influence. Since vaccination with humanized virus is more speedy in its effect than when bovine lymph is used, it is advisable to employ the former when readily obtainable and to make several insertions in order to increase the probability of success. Even a late vaccination in the stage of incubation may be of value, as it sometimes happens that this period lasts fourteen days or more. Early in the nineteenth century Waterhouse claimed that two days after infection vaccination would save the patient.

Good results from the subcutaneous injection of vaccine lymph have also been claimed by Farley and others, but the efficacy of this method of treatment appears to have been assumed rather than proven.

The speedy vaccination of all those who have been accidentally exposed to smallpox infection will do no harm, even if it fails to modify the disease when contracted.

Indeed, it is always advisable, since the persons exposed, even if not already infected, are liable to contract the disease through possible subsequent exposure; and in the case of a threatening epidemic no precaution should be neglected which might tend to lessen the number of possible cases.

Since no drug nor specific remedy exists which administered during the period of incubation will abort or modify the subsequent eruption, the only thing to be done is to prepare the patient by means of a rigid regimen and all possible hygienic measures to withstand the impending attack. When the fact of exposure is certain, forewarned should be forearmed.

Period of Invasion (Initial Stage).—At the outbreak of the initial symptoms of smallpox a correct diagnosis is rarely made, owing to the fact that headache, lumbar pain, chills, fever, and nausea are not sufficiently pathognomonic to always suggest the true nature of the disease. In those cases, however, where it is known that the patient has been exposed to infection and an attack of variola is consequently anticipated, the diagnosis is comparatively easy. In such a case the patient should be put to bed, or at least confined in a large, airy room, from which all draperies and superfluous articles, capable of absorbing infectious germs, should be at once removed. The temperature of the room should be kept as low as possible in summer and should not exceed 60° to 65° F. in winter. An extra bed or couch should be provided, to which the patient can make a convenient and agreeable change later in the course of the disease, especially if it proves to be of a severe type.

At the outset the bowels should be freely opened by a dose of calomel and soda, followed in the morning by a saline purgative; and since constipation is apt to persist in most cases throughout the course of the disease, it is advisable to administer a little cold citrate of magnesia or some other agreeable laxative from day to day.

A warm bath should be taken and the skin from head to foot thoroughly cleansed by vigorous soap friction and the application of an antiseptic lotion. If the disease proves mild, a daily bath can be taken; or when this does not seem advisable, the daily sponging of the whole body with cool water will usually lessen the fever and add greatly to the comfort of the sufferer. If the patient happens to belong to the class of the unvaccinated, or has not been vaccinated for many years, and there exists consequently the prospect of a severe attack, the hair and beard should be closely clipped. In most cases, however, this procedure can be left until the eruption has appeared, and if this is moderate in amount, the cutting of the hair, especially in the case of young girls and women, may not be necessary.

The diet, which throughout the course of smallpox is a matter of the greatest importance, should be light and nutritious during this stage, consisting mainly of milk, broth, or gruel.

The medicinal treatment of smallpox in this stage and throughout the course of the disease must be mainly symptomatic. Upon careful nursing and the prompt treatment of the various symptoms as they present themselves we must depend in great measure for the fortunate termination in any case. The remedies and special methods which have been vaunted by some as tending to abort or modify the eruption and to lessen the severity of the disease, have been tested by others and found wanting. A specific for variola comparable in its action to that of mercury in syphilis or quinine in malaria is at the present time unknown, although, in view of the recent advances in antitoxic medication, the discovery of such is a hope that may possibly be realized in the near future.

A high degree of fever in the initial stage of smallpox with intense headache and backache are symptoms which call loudly for relief, although they may not betoken a corresponding severity of the disease in its subsequent stages. Aconite, quinine, phenacetine, and other antipyretics are remedies which may now be advantageously given, and the daily cool bath, although it may not have the notable effect so often observed in typhoid fever, will assist in lowering the temperature.

If the fever is combined with extreme nervousness, the old and reliable Dover's powder will be found of service. In some cases delirium is present during the initial stage, and occasionally a suicidal tendency is manifested, which makes it necessary to have a watchful nurse in constant attendance upon the patient. Potassium bromide in full doses, chloral, or sulphonal may be advantageously employed as a sedative, but the most effective remedy is probably the hypodermic injection of the sulphate of morphine (gr. $\frac{1}{4}$).

If the headache, which is almost invariably present, is very severe, an ice-bag or cold cloth applied to the scalp will afford relief. The fear which has been entertained by some that such a procedure might tend to suppress the eruption is utterly groundless. For the lumbar pain, of which the patient often complains, a hot application will usually feel more grateful. The custom of applying mustard-plasters to the lower part of the back is not to be recommended, since the irritation of the skin which is caused thereby is liable to increase the eruption in that region and add to the subsequent discomfort of the patient. The theory that the eruption can be lessened upon the face by increasing the number of lesions upon some other part of the body has never proved successful in practice.

The sensation of thirst which is always present, and is often intolerable, can be alleviated by frequent sips of cold milk or by weak lemonade, either hot or cold. If there is extreme nausea and vomiting, as is usually the case with children, small pieces of ice dissolved in the mouth will relieve it together with the excessive thirst.

Period of Eruption.—With the outbreak of the papular eruption of smallpox, which usually appears upon the face on the third day of the disease, a notable decrease of the fever occurs with a decided improvement in the general condition of the patient. In a mild case, when a diagnosis of variola is not promptly made, the patient often returns to his business or pursues his or her customary duties with no thought of the danger to which others are exposed through contact or association. But the rapid development of the eruption soon leads to the discovery of its true nature and a realization of the importance of continued isolation.

During the papular and vesicular stage little or no internal medication is required, Gayton, an English writer on smallpox, who evidently shares the popular belief that the main duty of a physician is to give medicine, remarks that "we may also prescribe a little effervescing saline, for unless something is given in the form of medicine, the impression on the sick man's mind is that you are doing nothing to assist him." An intelligent public, in this country at least, is gradually awakening to the fact that skilful medical treatment cannot longer be measured by the number and size of the apothecaries' bottles.

Although the appetite may now return, a restriction of the diet to simple and nutritious articles of food, such as milk-toast, eggs, oysters, and jellies, should be enforced.

The daily bath should be continued, and there is no objection to its being made antiseptic by the addition of carbolic acid or bichloride of mercury. It is simpler and safer, however, to employ a plain bath and to disinfect the skin later by sponging with some antiseptic lotion, such as peroxide of hydrogen or permanganate of potassium. It has been claimed by some enthusiast, though never demonstrated, that carbolic soap will abort the disease.

The local treatment of the eruption during the papular and vesicular stage has been a subject of experimentation for centuries, and the prevailing opinion at the present time is that little or nothing can be done to arrest its development. Most of the local applications, like the mercurial and other plasters of former days, though doubtless of some value, have proved generally to be more uncomfortable than beneficial to the patient. Tincture of iodine, pure or diluted, with an equal part of alcohol, nitrate of silver solution, collodion, picric acid, and more recently ichthyol, have been advocated by some and rejected by others after a careful test of their merits. Gayton recommends the use of the old itch lotion of sulphur and quicklime when cases present themselves before eruption or during the papular stage. He claims that if the lotion is rubbed over the whole body every four or six hours it will prevent the papules from reaching the pustular stage and thus avert the severe secondary fever. This surprising statement he bases on the observation of hundreds of cases.

The effect of light upon the development of the smallpox eruption is a subject of considerable interest, and in recent years it has become one of therapeutic importance. As long ago as the fourteenth century John of Gaddesden and other physicians of his time were in the habit of excluding both light and fresh air from smallpox patients. The walls and furniture of the sick-room were painted red, on account of a peculiar virtue supposed to reside in this color, and the unfortunate occupant was nearly smothered by red curtains hung around his bed. Ever since that time it has been a common custom to darken the room of a smallpox patient, partly on account of the photophobia present during the course of the disease and partly on account of the idea that sunlight would aggravate the eruption. The fact that the face and hands are most intensely affected would seem to substantiate this idea, but the argument fails when we consider that the feet are usually the seat of an eruption scarcely less profuse.

It was claimed by Black, in 1867, that the complete exclusion of light from the eruption of smallpox, even when occurring in unvaccinated persons, effectually prevented pitting of the face. Barlow, Gallivardin, and others, have expressed a similar belief. Experimentation by Finsen, Unna, and others having demonstrated that it was not the heat of the sun but the ultra-violet or chemical rays which cause solar eczema and pigmentation of the skin, it was suggested by Finsen that in place of the complete exclusion of light in the treatment of variola, it was only necessary to eliminate the chemical rays of sunlight by means of red glass windows or red curtains. Acting upon this suggestion Lindholm, Svensen, Day, and others, treated smallpox by this new method, and made most favorable reports of their results. The red light proved agreeable and soothing to the eyes of the patients, frequently caused the vesicles to dry without becoming purulent, and lessened the suppurative fever. The patients, it is claimed, passed directly from the vesicular stage into convalescence, and neither pitting nor pigmentation of the skin was observed.

Some less enthusiastic experimenters with the red-light treatment of variola have been more moderate in their praises, and in some smallpox hospitals it has been tried and given up.

My own experience with this method is limited to the observation of a few cases treated at the Riverside Hospital in 1893. Under the direction of Dr. Cyrus Edson, health commissioner, one ward was fitted with red glass windows. The cases treated were of a mild type, and although no deaths occurred, the disease appeared to run its usual course and the experiment was negative as to results. In reply to a letter of inquiry, Dr. Edson writes me that "if the results had not been negative a very careful report would have been made." For the advancement of therapeutic knowledge it is indeed unfortunate that while the enthusiast is always so ready to write, the sceptic or unsuccessful experimenter is usually inclined to remain silent.

Period of Suppuration.—With the transformation of the smallpox vesicles into pustules a rise of temperature occurs which is commonly known as the "secondary fever," and in severe cases the swelling of the face, hands, and feet usually occasions the most intense suffering. The chief dangers of this stage arise from the possibility of septic poisoning and the probability of a greater or less degree of exhaustion.

A nutritious diet is now of the utmost importance, and in severe cases bouillon, malted milk, or other prepared foods which can be readily swallowed should be given every two or three hours. If the patient is in a stupor, he may be awakened in order to receive the necessary nourishment, but the calm, refreshing sleep which sometimes follows a period of wakefulness and complete exhaustion should not be disturbed. Alcoholic stimulants are usually of great service in this stage and may be given freely, especially at night and in the early morning hours when the patient's vitality is at its lowest ebb. In case of delirium, rectal alimentation will often be found necessary as a substitute for or a supplement to oral feeding. The rectum should first be thoroughly cleansed by an enema of soap and water and then from four to six ounces of milk and brandy or eggnog may be injected.

As the eruption of smallpox attacks the mucous membrane of the mouth, nose, and throat, as well as the skin, difficulty in swallowing and considerable discomfort in breathing is often present, especially during the suppurative stage. If the patient is able to sit up and gargle, peroxide of hydrogen or some other antiseptic solution should be used at regular and frequent intervals. In case of extreme prostration, when any effort by the patient or the mere raising of the head might lead to syncope or symptoms of collapse, it is advisable to wash out the patient's throat and nostrils with a large swab of absorbent cotton, dipped in a saturated solution of boric acid. Pyrozone, borolyptol, listerine, and other liquids may be conveniently used for this purpose diluted with one or two parts of water. Small pieces of ice or ice-cream given at frequent intervals with a small coffeespoon will usually be found extremely grateful to the suffering patient.

For a purulent conjunctivitis which may sometimes result from the presence of pustules on the lids, the saturated solution of boric acid should be frequently used in the form of a spray.

When delirium occurs in this stage the patient must be closely watched, and, if necessary, the limbs may be kept quiet by linen sheets folded and carried across the bed and fastened at either end. Since chloral given by the mouth is liable to cause œdema of the glottis, it may be advantageously administered by the rectum, or in its place the bromides or a hypodermic injection of sulphate of morphine may be substituted, although when the patient is suffering at the same time from severe bronchitis the use of opium is objectionable.

The treatment of the eruption in the suppurative stage is of the greatest importance so far as the comfort of the patient is concerned. A host of applications and peculiar methods of treatment have been recommended and tested in successive epidemics. Many of these have been found to have no effect save to intensify the patient's horrible appearance and to aggravate his discomfort. From time immemorial attempts have been made to prevent the pitting of the face after the disease by treatment of the individual lesions. The cauterization of the pustules with nitrate of silver after evacuation of the pus—the so-called ectrotic method—has been practised by many in the past, but the consensus of opinion at the present day seems to be that the procedure is as useless as it is painful. The ointments, plasters, pastes, and varnishes which have also been advocated are usually unpleasant or troublesome to use, and in the pustular stage are not likely to accomplish any desirable end. At this period it is too late to consider the possibility of preventing pitting, although the resulting injury to the skin may be reduced to a minimum by the use of all local measures which tend to reduce the grade of inflammation.

For the highly inflamed condition of the skin which characterizes the suppurative stage of smallpox, especially in its confluent form, cold water is, beyond all doubt, the best antiphlogistic. The cold compresses advocated years ago by Hebra constitute the simplest method of local treatment and one which is most grateful and beneficial to the patient. They exclude the air, macerate and soften the lesions, and lessen the local inflammation. Although it cannot be claimed that they modify in any degree the development and course of the eruption, it is doubtful whether anything better in the way of local treatment has ever been suggested. Pieces of lint should be dipped in cold water and applied smoothly to the face and other portions of the body where the eruption is abundant and the skin inflamed. To prevent their drying too rapidly a little glycerine may be added to the water and the lint covered with gutta-percha tissue or oiled silk. Moore recommends covering the face with a light mask of lint and oiled silk, having holes for the eyes, nose, and mouth. The lint is wet with a mixture of glycerin and iced water (fʒi-fʒi). If preferred, a cold solution of boric acid may be used in place of plain water, and when there is an excessive and unpleasant odor present, thymol may be added to the solution. Immermann states that he used for a time sublimate dressings to the face (1–1000), but found that plain water did quite as much good and was safer to use.

Next to the face, the hands and feet suffer most from the eruption of smallpox, and, owing to the fact that the skin is not as lax in the latter region, particularly upon the fingers and toes, the inflammatory swelling of these parts is always attended with extreme pain when pustules are numerous. Under such conditions it may be found advisable, in place of merely wrapping the hands and feet in lint and oiled silk, to immerse them in pans or pails of water, or to supply the patient with mittens and stockings made of vulcanized rubber cloth. Indeed, if the patient is not in too critical a condition, he may be immersed for hours in a bath, as recommended by Hebra for the treatment of extensive burns, pemphigus, and various ulcerating affections involving a large portion of the body.

Period of Dessication.—When the distended, semi-globular pustules begin to dry, they tend to flatten, and often undergo a secondary umbilication from the shriveling of the central portion of the pock. In favorable cases the general condition of the patient improves as the fever subsides, and a more substantial diet may now be allowed.

The symptom which usually causes most local discomfort at this stage is the itching which invariably accompanies the drying of the pustules. This is often intolerable, and much of the pitting left after an attack of smallpox may be due to the tearing of the crusts from the face and other parts.

The best application which can now be made to the skin for the double purpose of softening the crusts and allaying the pruritus is a solution of carbolic acid in olive oil (five or ten per cent.). When the itching sensation of the face and hands is intense, it can be greatly relieved if the nurse will frequently spray these parts with pure chloroform, or, if the crusts have an unpleasant odor, with a mixture of chloroform and some antiseptic solution.

In the case of restless or unmanageable children the elbows may be put in splints so that the finger-nails cannot come in contact with the face.

Period of Convalescence.—When the crusts have dried and fallen from the face and body and no unpleasant complications still exist, the patient may be considered as a convalescent. No treatment is now required except a liberal diet, the daily bath, and a continued application of carbolized vaseline or some antiseptic oil. When the discolored cicatrices left after the falling of the crusts appear elevated and hard, as is frequently the case upon the face and hands (variola verrucosa), it is customary with some to paint them with tincture of iodine. A pleasanter and more effective application is a twenty per cent. solution of resorcin in rose-water.

When the skin has assumed its normal smoothness, and no indication of the disease remains except the dull purplish-red spots where the crusts have fallen, the patient may be regarded as well, and, after a careful disinfection of his body, he may be furnished with fresh or thoroughly disinfected clothing and discharged from the hospital or sick-room.

In disinfecting a patient prior to his discharge, not only should a prolonged bath be taken, but the head should be thoroughly shampooed with carbolic soap, the nails cut and scrubbed with the same, and the mucous orifices of the body cleansed with peroxide of hydrogen.

Prophylactic Treatment.—The prophylactic treatment of smallpox is of vastly more importance than any therapeutic measure, since it concerns a community and not merely an individual. In dealing with smallpox cases many physicians discover only too late that an ounce of prevention is worth many pounds of cure. When a case of smallpox is first recognized, or even suspected, the patient should be isolated in a room from which all unnecessary articles of furniture, especially of soft texture, have been removed. A sheet moistened with some volatile disinfectant should be hung before the door, and no one allowed to enter the room save the nurse and doctor. A change of clothing should be made outside by the former whenever leaving the room, and a gown should be ready for the latter to wear at each visit. Upon leaving the sick-room the physician should carefully disinfect his hands and remain for some time in the fresh air before making another call. When the diagnosis is positively made, all who have come in contact with the patient, unless manifestly immune, should be found and vaccinated without delay.

During the course of the disease all discharges, such as fæces, urine, sputa, or vomited matter, should be received in glass or earthen vessels containing a five per cent. solution of carbolic acid. Handkerchiefs and soiled rags should be burned or with towels and soiled sheets placed in a carbolic solution and allowed to remain for twelve hours. The plates, knives, forks, and spoons used by the patient should be kept in the sick-room and washed in a disinfectant solution by the nurse, while any uneaten food should be treated in the same manner as the patient's discharges. When the patient has fully recovered, and, after personal disinfection, has left the sick-room, this should be thoroughly fumigated. The mattress and bed-coverings should be burned or, in large cities, sent to the Board of Health for disinfection. In case of death the corpse should be washed with a strong bichloride solution or painted with carbolized oil (twenty per cent.), and buried or cremated as quickly as possible. The clothing worn by the patient at the beginning of the disease should be destroyed or disinfected by baking for an hour in an oven at a temperature of 220° F., or steamed for five minutes at a temperature of 212° F.

In disinfecting the sick-room, the furniture, woodwork, and floor should first be scrubbed with carbolic soap and hot water or a solution of bichloride of mercury (1–500). The windows, ventilators, and fireplace should then be tightly closed and the fumes of burning sulphur or formaldehyde gas used to complete the disinfection. Sublimed sulphur burned in a moist atmosphere (one pound to every thousand cubic feet of space) is effective, but is at the same time objectionable on account of its tendency to bleach or discolor all textile fabrics. In well-furnished rooms, containing articles liable to be injured by sulphur or steam, such as wall-paper, paintings, books, etc., it is advisable to use, whenever possible, a formaldehyde gas-generator, which can usually be obtained from the local Board of Health.

CHAPTER IV.

VACCINATION consists in the inoculation of virus taken from the pock produced by vaccinia.

Vaccine Virus.—Virus has been taken from vaccine vesicles on almost all animals susceptible to vaccinia, but throughout the greater part of the last century the material used in the vaccination of human subjects was taken generally from a vaccine vesicle on the arm of a previously unvaccinated healthy child. Such virus when collected at the proper time was found to take with great regularity, and vesicles resulting from its use were uniformly well developed and typical. Humanized virus was, however, open to the objection that it could communicate disease if the child were not perfectly healthy, and as a matter of fact it did communicate syphilis in a certain number of instances. The possibility of this infection was so serious an objection to the use of virus from this source that in the last quarter of the century calf virus, recommended and used in Italy many years before, was gradually substituted for human virus, and at the present time the use of animal virus is general in Europe and in the United States. In the production of virus, calves are for commercial reasons generally preferred to other animals. Calves take typically, and a large amount of virus can be collected from them, whereas all other animals either are comparatively expensive, or take poorly, or are able to furnish but little virus. Cows also are more expensive, are less easily handled, and develop vaccine vesicles less typically.

In the practical production of vaccine virus calves are vaccinated much as human beings are vaccinated, but over a larger area. Usually the posterior abdomen and the insides of the thighs are covered with superficial linear incisions, and into these incisions the seed virus is rubbed. In the laboratory of the New York City Health Department all operations relating to the vaccination of the animals and to the collection of the virus are carried on in an operating-room provided with a cement floor, glazed brick walls, and equipped with enamelled metal operating furniture, such as would be used in a hospital. The attendants wear sterile gowns and the technique of the operations is aseptic. The seed virus is either humanized virus collected by touching sterile pieces of bone to the serum exuding from ruptured vesicles on the arms of children, or in the great majority of cases bovine glycerinated virus which has been preserved two months or longer.

It is found that the crust of the vesicle, the serum issuing from the vesicle after the crust is removed, the pulp which forms the semi-solid contents and base of the vesicle, and the serum which exudes from the base of the vesicle after the pulp has been removed by a curette, all convey material capable of producing the vaccine vesicle in a susceptible person, and are therefore all different forms of vaccine virus. It has been shown, however, that if any of this material is filtered, so that all the solid particles are removed, the filtrate is inefficient. In other words, the serum is efficient as vaccine virus simply by virtue of the solid particles which it contains. It is also found that the pulp is so rich in the active principle of vaccine virus that it may be mixed with several times its weight of glycerin or other diluent and still maintain its efficiency.

The different sorts of vaccine virus on the market are simply different ways of supplying this material coming from the vesicle. Most material is in one of three forms,—

(*a*) The pulp diluted with some excipient, such as glycerin, vaseline, or lanolin. The emulsion, made by mixture with glycerin, may be contained in a vial or in a capillary tube, or may rest on some holder, such as an ivory or bone point. In the latter case the point is usually protected by some form of cap. Mixture with vaseline or lanolin makes a paste, which is usually issued in a box. This is in use in parts of Italy and in India.

(*b*) The serum dried on a holder, as an ivory or bone point or a quill.

(*c*) The serum mixed with some excipient, usually solid or semi-solid, until it becomes a paste, and furnished like dried serum on a holder.

For a physician the choice among these three forms is governed by considerations of efficiency, safety, and ease of use. All the forms are under certain conditions efficient, but comparative tests show that the emulsion of the pulp issued by different laboratories is much more certainly efficient than the other forms, and the glycerinated emulsion is at present in most general use both abroad and in this country.

It is also true that all forms may be perfectly safe. All forms contain bacteria when prepared, and the majority of these bacteria die within a few weeks or months after preparation. On account of the mildly antiseptic quality of glycerin the bacteria in the glycerinated emulsion usually die sooner than those in the other forms of virus, and so far as bacteria are objectionable in the virus the glycerinated form may therefore be said to be somewhat preferable. It should be added, however, both that glycerinated virus is usually put in the market before the bacteria have disappeared and that the bacteria present in virus issued by well-conducted laboratories are not found to be pathogenic to persons when inoculated by the customary method of vaccination.

The ease of use of any form of virus depends largely upon the custom of the physician. In vaccinating a large number at one time there can be no question that the use of a liquid virus supplied in vials is more rapid than the use of a dried virus, as the latter has to be thoroughly moistened before it can be applied effectively.

Methods of Vaccination.—The usual method of vaccination is to scarify a spot on the skin and to rub the virus on that spot. The choice of place depends partly on æsthetic reasons and partly on convenience. To avoid the formation of an unsightly scar on the arm, the leg may be used instead. If the arm is chosen, the insertion of the deltoid is the place of election on account of the small number of lymphatics there. If the leg is chosen, the area just below the head of the fibula presents the same anatomical advantage; but a spot a short distance above the knee on the outside of the thigh is often thought to offer less opportunity for injury and infection. Choice between the sides depends in an adult on the use to which the vaccinated limb is to be put, and in a baby on the advantage of vaccinating the side which is carried away from the nurse.

The size of the scarification is important. The vesicle is always somewhat larger than the scarification, and the larger the vesicle the greater danger that the surface may be broken, and the more opportunity there is for the introduction of extraneous infection. A spot as large as the head of a medium pin is about as small as can be easily scarified, and vesicles formed on such scarifications are least liable to have inflammatory complications. If, as certain evidence tends to show, a larger area of scar guarantees greater protection, and if a larger area is therefore desired, it is better to vaccinate in two or three small spots than in one large one. It is somewhat difficult to rub the virus from a bone point on a spot of the minute size described, and as this form of virus is usually more dilute than glycerinated virus, a larger area may safely be employed.

The scarification may be made with any sharp instrument, or with the point itself. The only precaution necessary is that the instrument should be free from infection. As a scarifier the ordinary cambric needle presents the advantages that it is usually clean, is easily sterilized, and is so inexpensive that a fresh one can be used for every operation.

It is not necessary that the scarification should draw blood, although blood is not objectionable unless it flows so freely as to wash away the virus, or unless the subject has hæmophilia.

Although with a notably susceptible subject or with especially active virus it may be sufficient simply to smear the virus on the scarified area, it is usually necessary and always advisable to rub in the virus with a wooden slip or with the point firmly and thoroughly.

Other methods of introducing vaccine virus are by puncture, by deep injection, and by the mouth.

In the method by puncture either a grooved lancet or a hollow needle may be used. A shallow puncture is made and the virus is deposited in it. The resulting vesicle is usually small and nearly circular, and generally remains free from infection; but as the hole in which the virus is placed is small, it is possible that the issuing blood may wash it away completely, and the percentage of success with this method of inoculation is not quite so large, even in careful hands, as by the process of scarification with the same virus. Animal experiments with deep injection of virus through a hypodermic syringe and with administration of virus by the mouth show that there is no certainty of successful vaccination by these means, and that when success results there is no proof of it without a subsequent vaccination on the skin to test or to demonstrate the immunity.

Care after Vaccination.—As vaccination is a surgical procedure, it should be conducted aseptically with a sterile instrument on clean skin, and the wound should be guarded against extraneous infection. It is well therefore to put either a sterile gauze cover or a clean shield over the wound as soon as the virus has been sufficiently absorbed, and to leave the protection on until the natural crust has been formed,—*i.e.*, for a few hours. If the guard could be kept in position without motion and also without injurious pressure, it might remain until the process ended with the formation of a scar and the exfoliation of the crust; but practically it is so certain that the guard will be moved that it is wise to remove it and to trust to the protection of a clean muslin or linen cloth attached to the loose sleeve or other undergarment. For a day or two at the time when the inflammation is at its height it may be well again to guard by a shield against injury from a blow or push, but the shield should always be regarded as itself a danger. If by any accident the vaccine pustule becomes infected, it should be treated like any other infected wound,—the crust removed, the ulcer cleansed with antiseptics and dressed surgically. The immunity given by the pock is not at all lessened by this treatment.

Normal Clinical Course.—After primary vaccination in man there is a stage of incubation lasting for from forty-eight to seventy-two hours; a papule then develops, and by the end of the third or fourth day this has begun to show umbilication and a vesicular structure. When fully developed, about the sixth day after vaccination, the vesicle is distended and pearly in color. On the seventh or eighth day the areola develops,—*i.e.*, the skin about the vesicle becomes hard, sensitive, and red, the redness extending a variable distance, not usually more than two inches from the edge of the vesicle. In the course of the next day or two the vesicle loses its pearly appearance and becomes opaque and often slightly yellow. With the development of the areola and of the pustule the adjacent lymph glands may swell and become somewhat painful; there may also be constitutional derangement,—some fever, pain, anorexia, restlessness, and more or less prostration; there is usually a moderate leucocytosis. About the eleventh or twelfth day the areola begins to fade, the constitutional symptoms to subside, and the pustule to dry up. A dark crust is formed which drops off usually between the eighteenth and twenty-fifth days, leaving a rosy depressed scar on which not infrequently a secondary scab is formed, to be shed a few days later.

Variations in the Clinical Course.—The vesicles may appear on the second day, but it is more frequently delayed until the fourth, fifth, sixth, seventh, or even the eighth day, and cases have been observed in which the delay was even longer.

The areola, which should be bright red, may be purple, and may extend a long distance from the vesicle.

The pustule may be hemorrhagic or may be filled with greenish pus; in this case there is probably a mixed infection.

Sometimes instead of a vesicle there appears a hard elevated nodule, in color like a red raspberry. With this there is usually no areola, and no constitutional symptoms develop. The growth is usually an evidence of poor virus. It may persist for some time before absorption.

The course may be abortive,—*i.e.*, the vesicle does not develop completely; pustulation comes early and the crust is shed and the scar formed before the end of the second week. This course is normal though not invariable in revaccinations.

The scar may be poorly marked, even when the vaccination has run a typical course.

Complications.—The most frequent complications are infections and eruptions. An infection may be, of course, of many sorts. It may be, for example, the streptococcus of erysipelas, or the bacillus of tetanus, but it is oftenest a skin coccus. These infections may be introduced with the virus, with the instrument, or later through wounds in the vesicle or pustule. Erysipelas and tetanus following vaccination are exceedingly rare, and it has never been shown that in a case of tetanus the germ was inoculated at the time of vaccination.

Eruptions are probably usually due to a chemical irritation produced by the development of the vaccinia; they are analogous to the eruptions following the injection of antitoxine and the ingestion of various drugs. They vary in appearance, sometimes resemble the eruption of measles or of scarlet fever, and again are urticarial; they are macular, papular, and vesicular.

When a moist eczema is present there may be auto-inoculation of the pock on the affected area and a general confluent vaccine eruption appear.

Immunity.—The immunity against smallpox, or vaccinia, produced by vaccination is of gradual growth, and is not complete until the period of suppuration, about the beginning of the second week. Natural immunity is said to exist, and is probable, but it is exceedingly rare. Vaccination of a pregnant woman rarely, if ever, confers immunity on the fœtus.

Duration of Immunity.—Sometimes a single vaccination gives immunity for life. Usually, however, susceptibility returns at latest seven to ten years after vaccination, and the second vaccination may give immunity for the rest of the lifetime, or susceptibility may return again and again. Failure of active, properly inserted virus shows only that the person so vaccinated is at that time immune, but conveys absolutely no information about the condition a few months later. The appearance of the scar is not a trustworthy guide as to immunity. Susceptibility to vaccination returns frequently within one year, and has returned in three months from the time of a successful vaccination. Susceptibility to smallpox probably returns, as a rule, later than susceptibility to vaccinia. It is rare that a case even of varioloid occurs within five years of a successful vaccination.

Conclusions.—Every child should be vaccinated at the time of election during the first year of life, and should be revaccinated before beginning school-life with its possibility of exposure. Every person, no matter at what age, should be vaccinated at a time of possible exposure to smallpox unless he has been successfully vaccinated within three months.

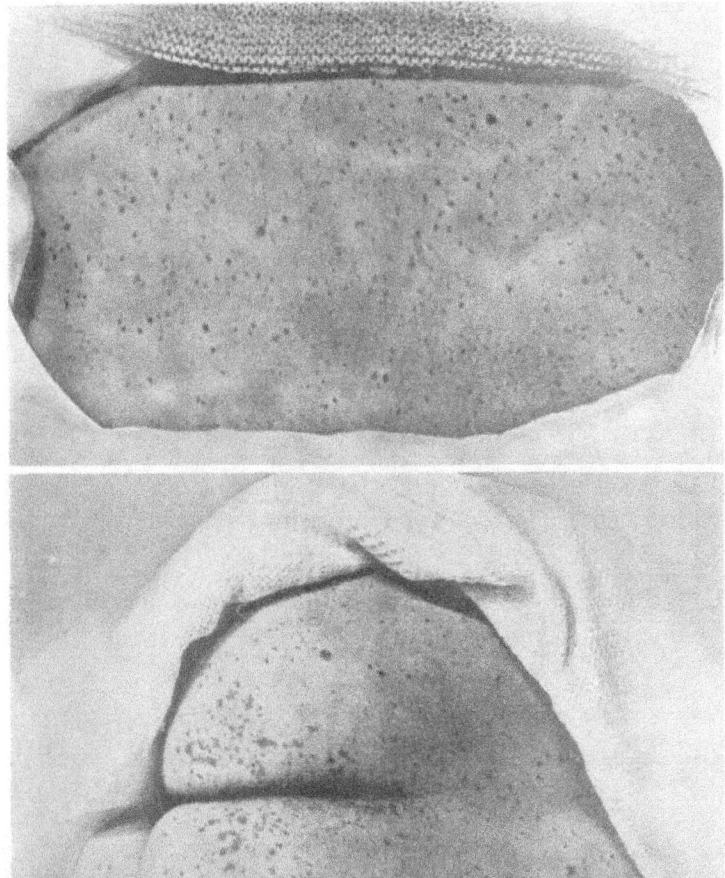

VARIOLA ERYTHEMATOSA.
(First day of eruption).

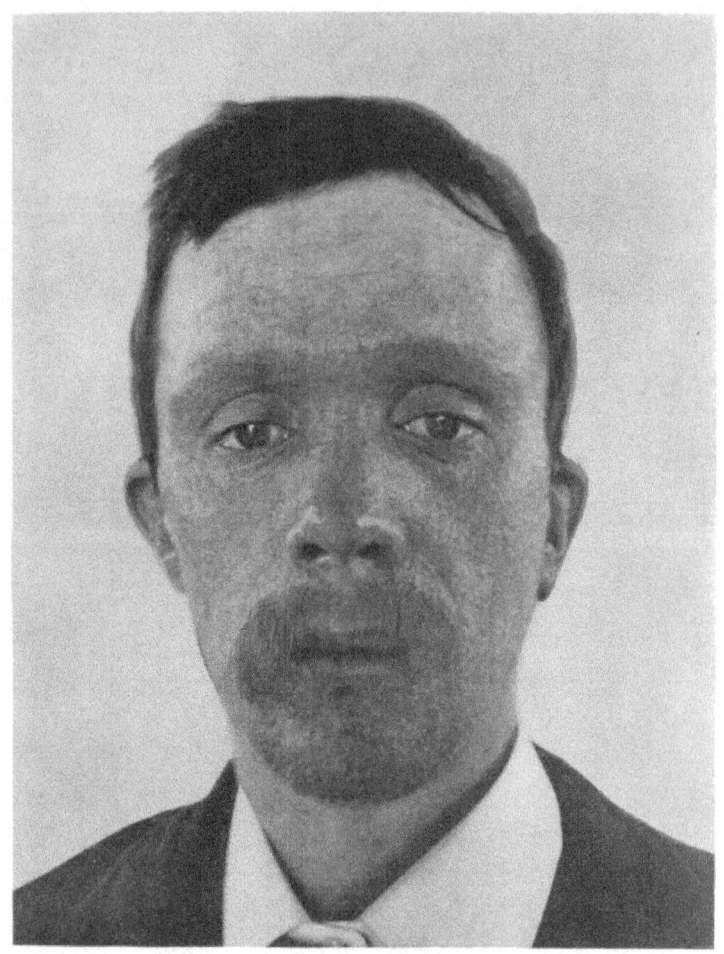

VARIOLA PAPULOSA.
(Second day).

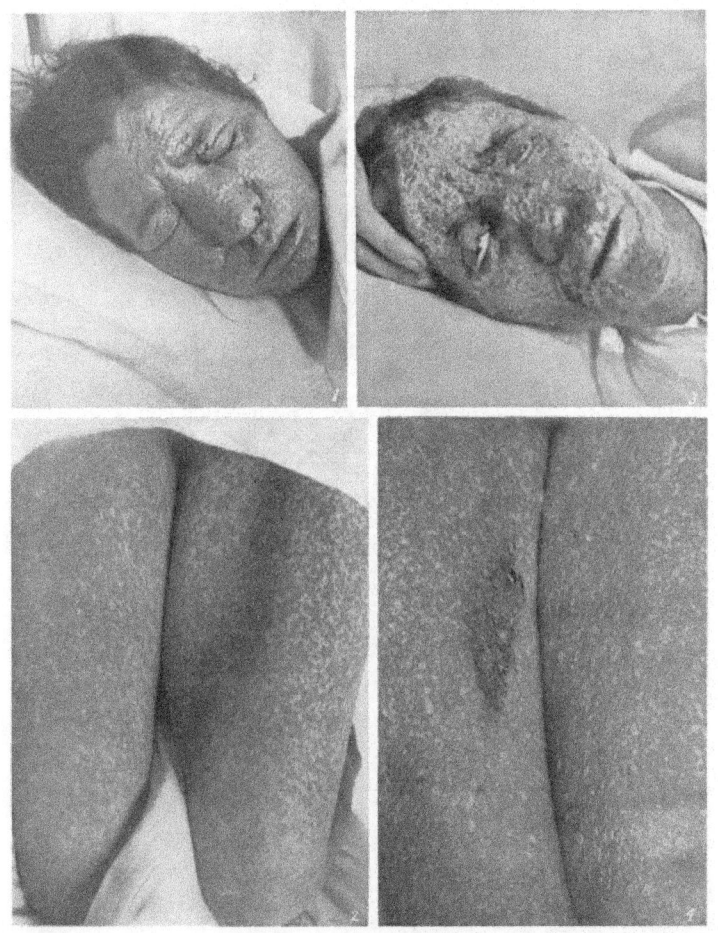

VARIOLA HEMORRHAGICA.
(Second day—Fourth day).

37

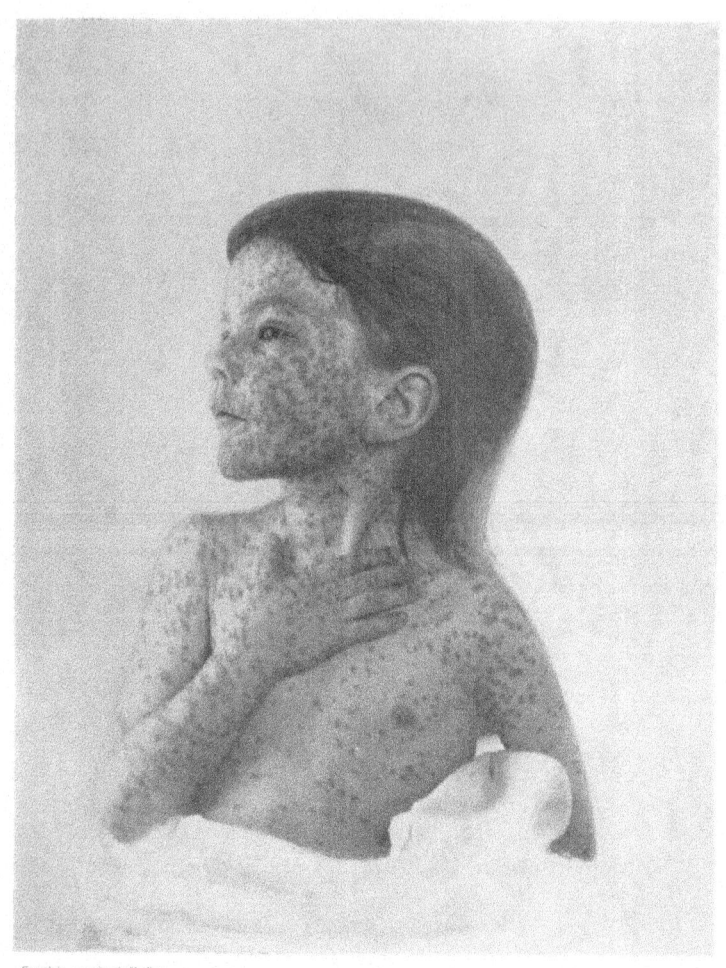

VARIOLA VESICULOSA.
(Fourth day).

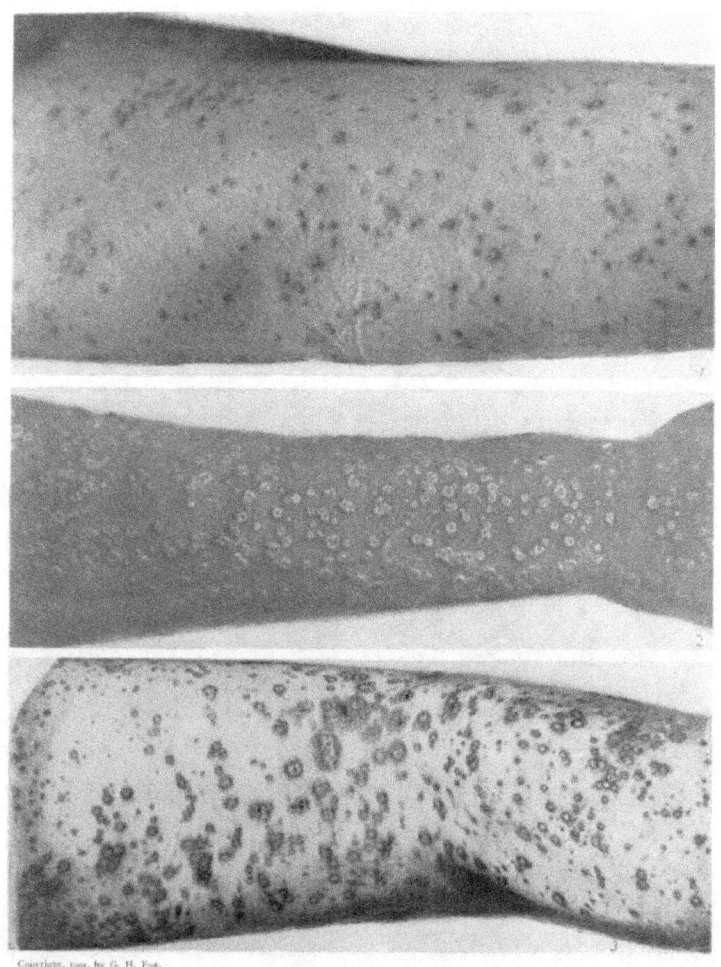

VARIOLA VESICULOSA.
(Third day—Fifth day—Sixth day).

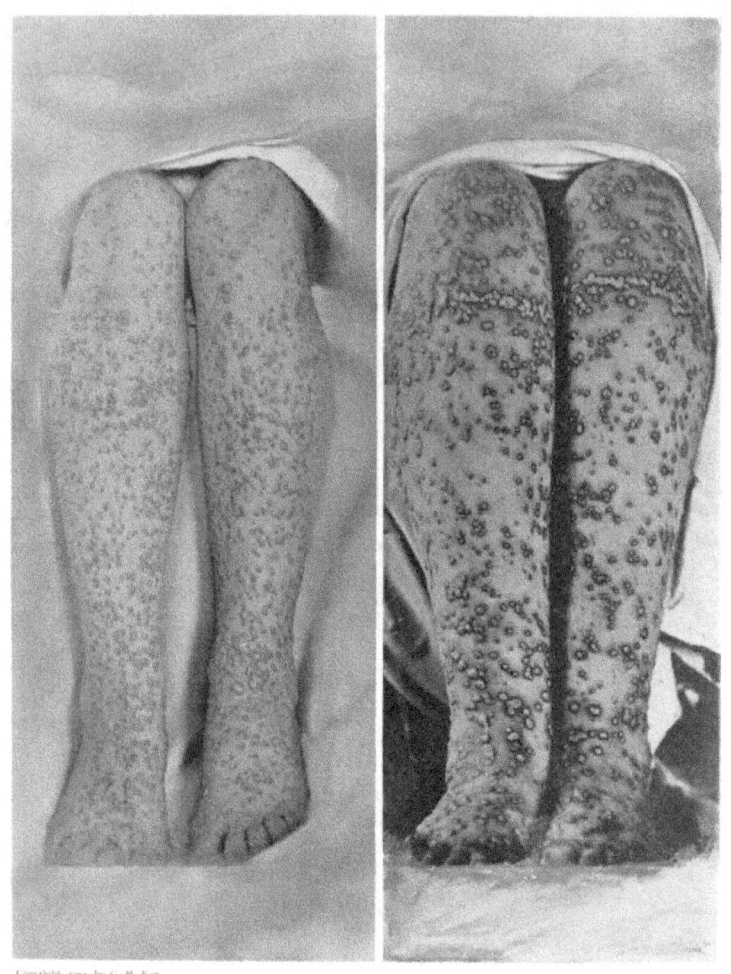

VARIOLA SEMI-CONFLUENS.
(Fifth day—Sixth day).

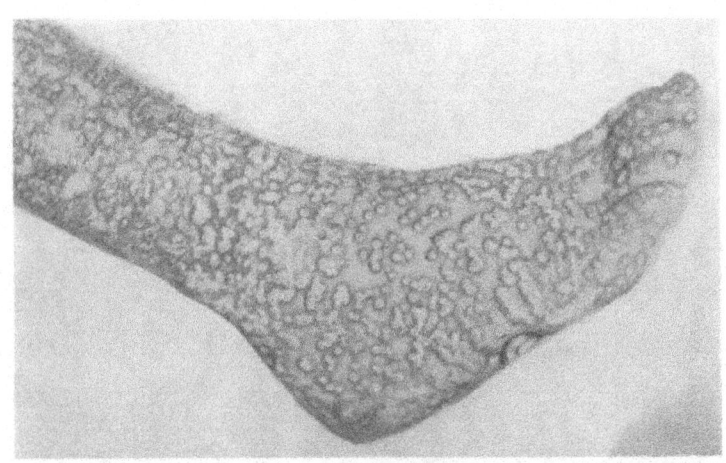

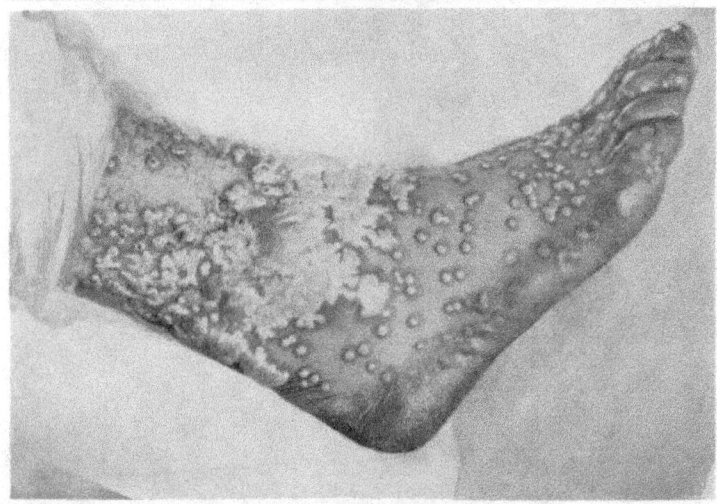

VARIOLA CONFLUENS.
(Seventh day—Eighth day).

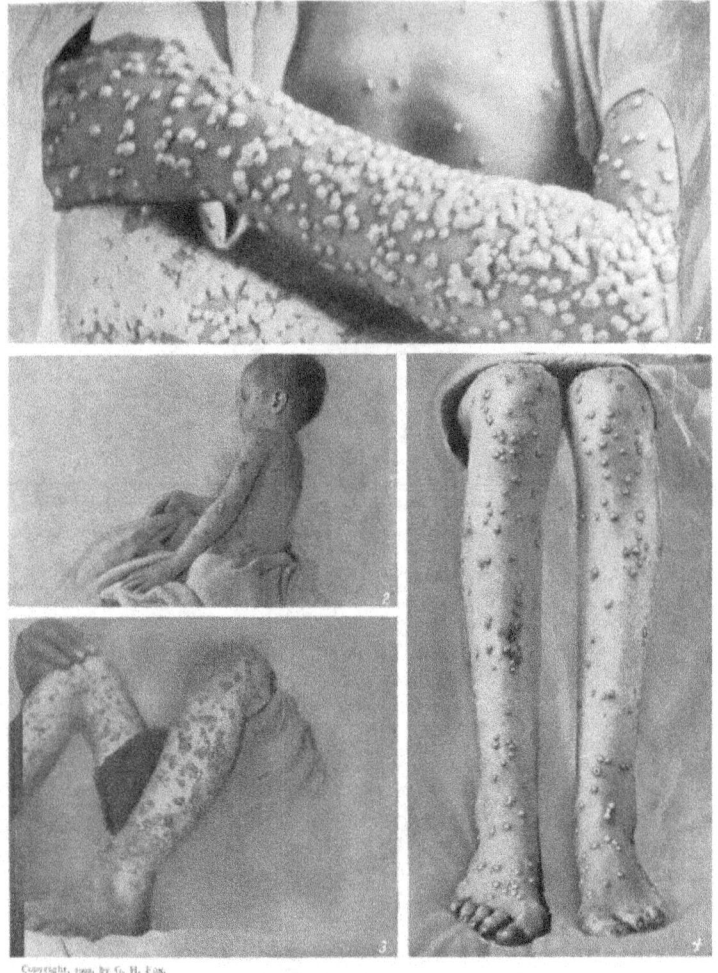

VARIOLA PUSTULOSA.
(Ninth day).

42

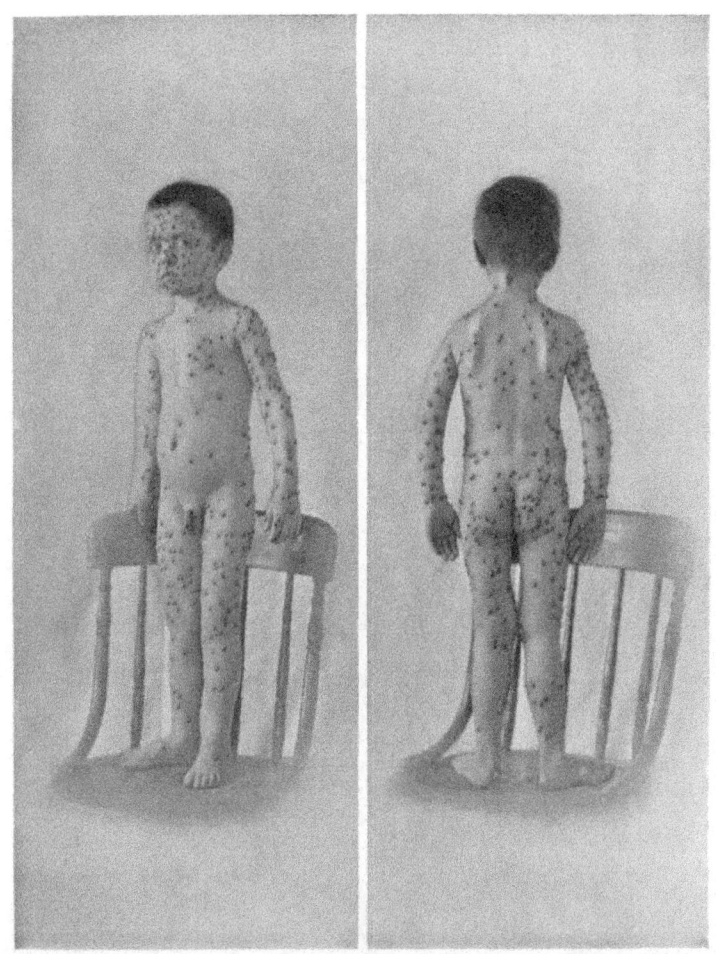

VARIOLA DISCRETA.
(Ninth day).

43

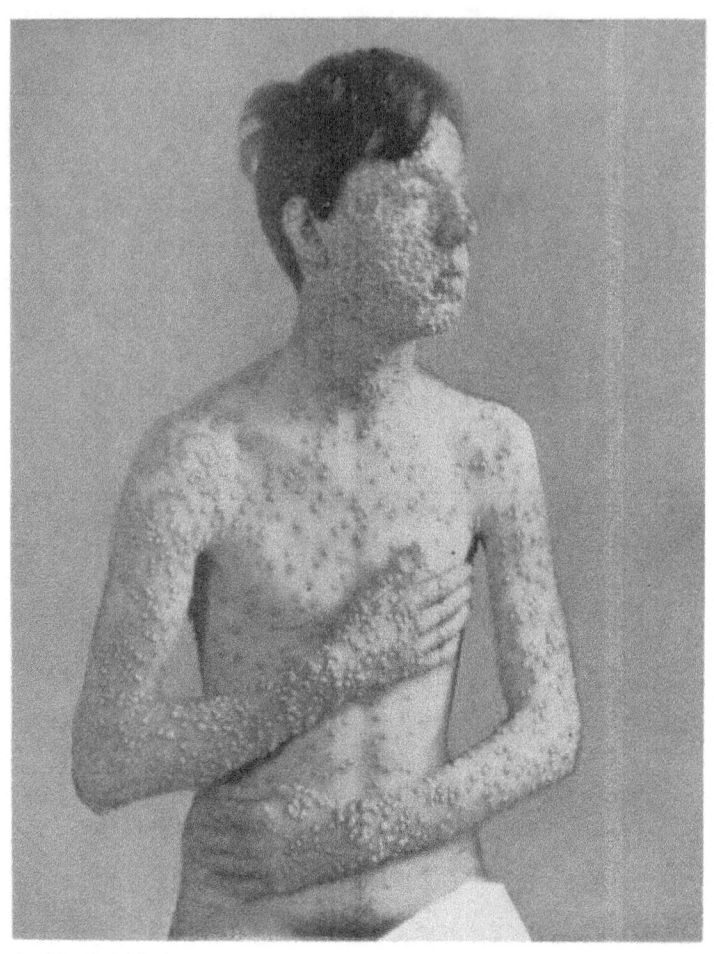

VARIOLA PUSTULOSA.
(Tenth day).

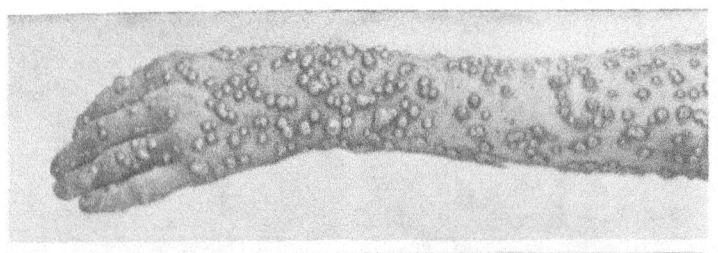

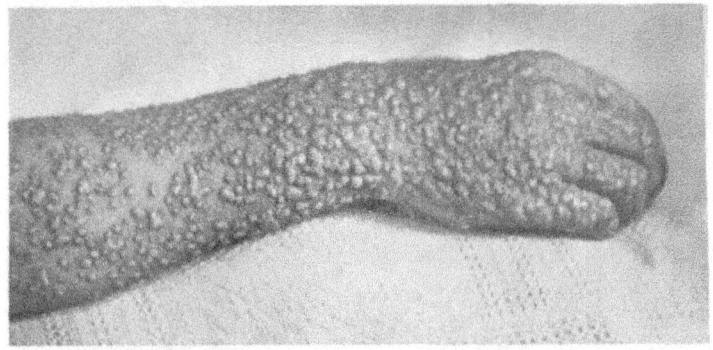

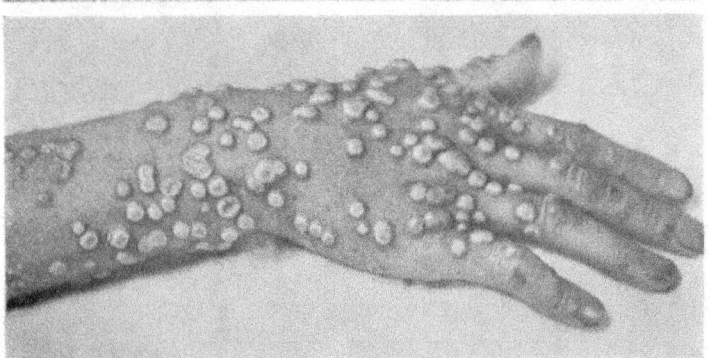

VARIOLA PUSTULOSA.
(Ninth day—Tenth day—Eleventh day).

45

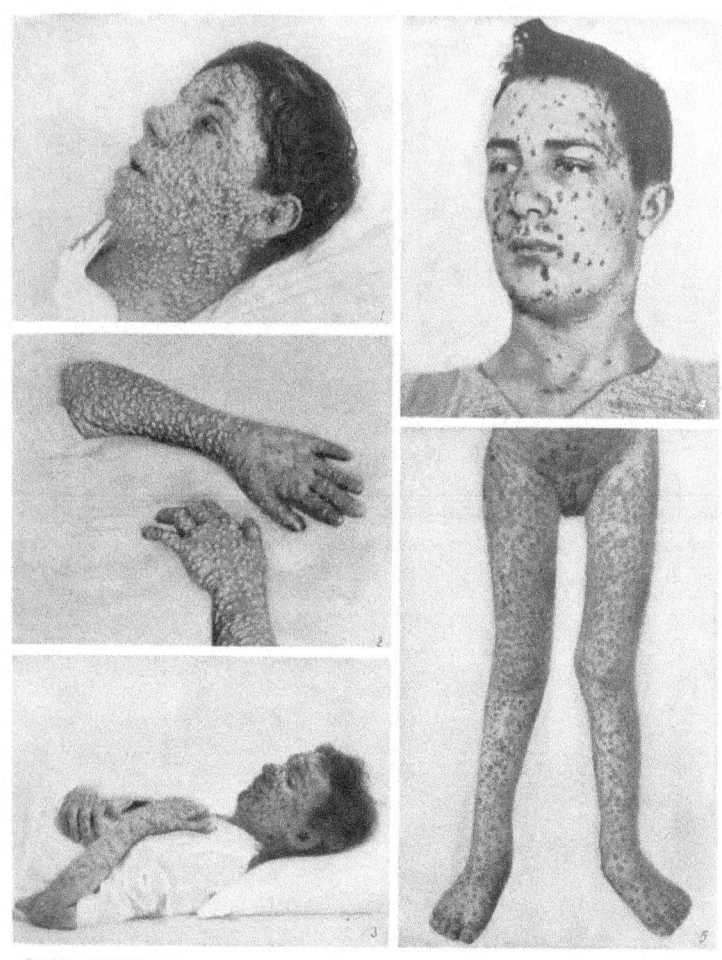

VARIOLA PUSTULOSA ET CRUSTOSA.
(Tenth day—Twelfth day).

46

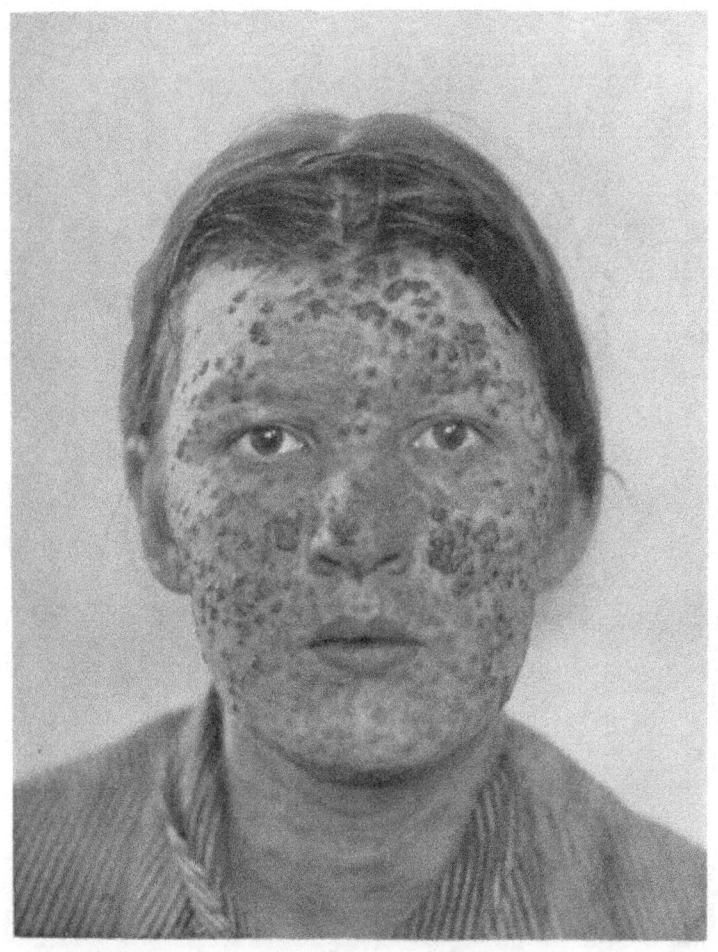

VARIOLA CRUSTOSA.
(Eighteenth day).

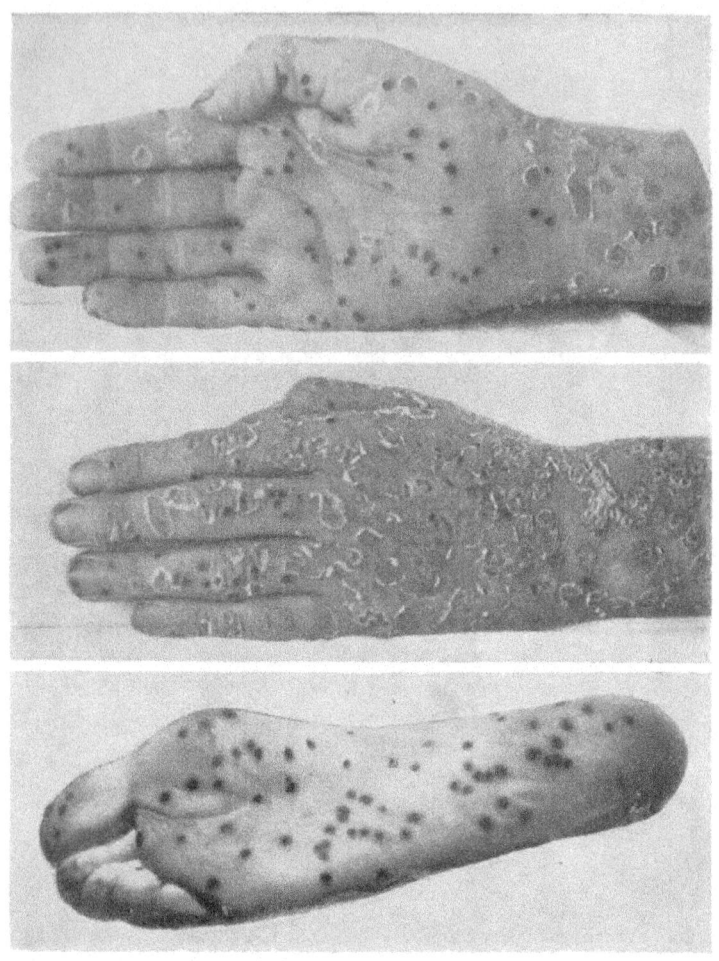

VARIOLA DESICCATA ET SQUAMOSA.
(Twentieth day).

48

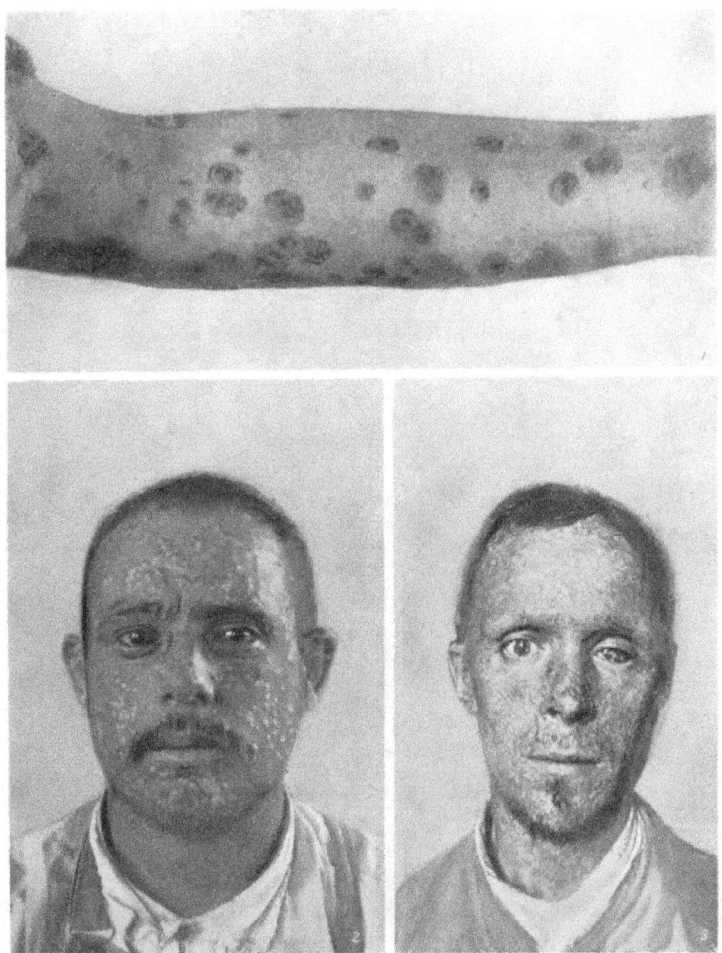

1. PIGMENTATION AFTER VARIOLA. (30th day).
2. VERRUCOUS SCARS. (25th day).   3. CONFLUENT PITTING. (35th day).

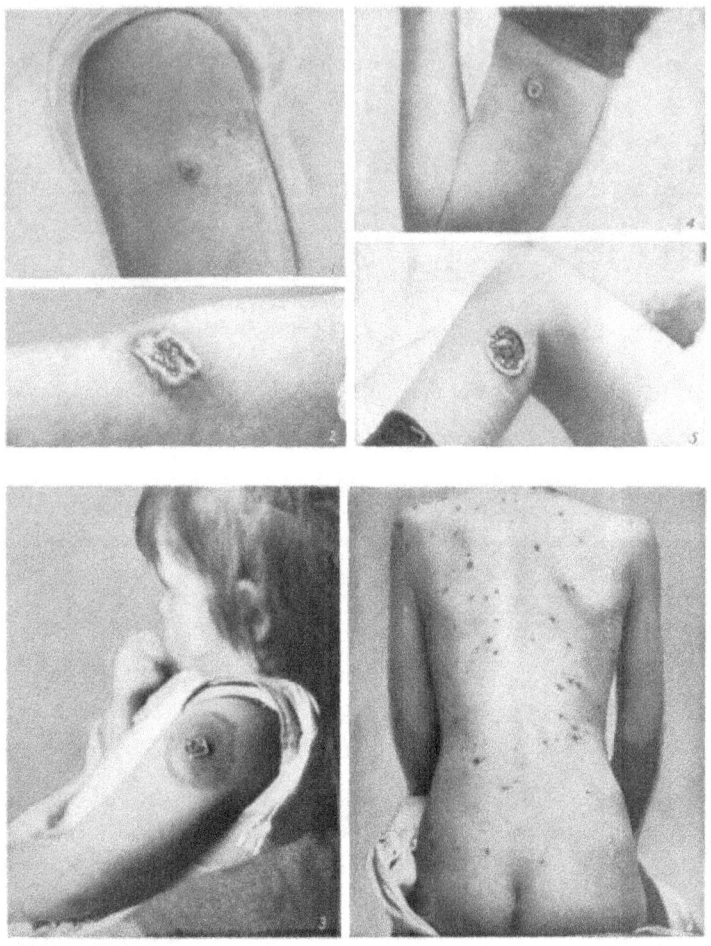

1. VACCINIA. (4th day).
2. VACCINIA. (8th day).
3. PRIMARY VACCINATION. (8th day).
4. VACCINIA. (8th day).
5. VACCINATION ULCER.
6. VARICELLA. (3d day).